# Reveal the Best in You!

by

## Isela Garcia

authorHOUSE™

1663 LIBERTY DRIVE, SUITE 200
BLOOMINGTON, INDIANA 47403
(800) 839-8640
WWW.AUTHORHOUSE.COM

First published by AuthorHouse 09/23/05

ISBN: 1-4208-5207-8 (sc)

Printed in the United States of America
Bloomington, Indiana

This book is printed on acid-free paper.

Illustrator: Rosa D. Aguilar

My deep love and appreciation to my children, Franchesca, Ernesto, Armida, for their total support and encouragement.

# Table of Contents

# Getting it Together!

Hello, my name is Isela Garcia, and I want to welcome you to read and enjoy my book. When you have finished, believe in what is taught to you, and then resign yourself to one of the suggestions, and practice to learn it for your own benefit. Let me guide and teach you to reach some or your full potential. Take your time, and with a clear mind and a little determination, you will notice a refreshing change in the way you feel in some or all parts of your body.

This book will hopefully be more rewarding in other aspects because you will take notice of your personality, character, looks and inner self.

Thank you!

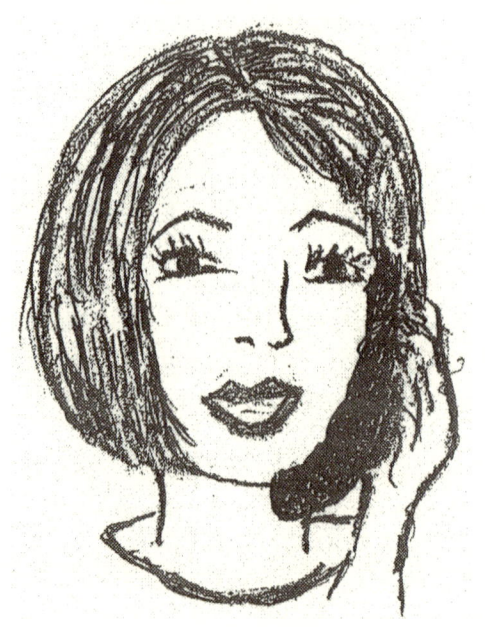

# Basic training

Let me begin in an area we are all familiar with...using the telephone. This is a utensil that is very much taken for granted. We feel lost without it. It expresses the reputation at home, business or any organization in how a person answers the telephone. People can tell about you or the company you represent, just by listening to the sound of your voice. A friendly greeting is a reflection of you, it should reveal eagerness to assist them. Keep in mind, these callers are seeking information, so put yourself in their place. Help them and they will love it. You will make their day and yours.

An example: you call a relative and ask how they are doing. They answer with a cold flat response, "fine", and not ask how you are doing. Instead they say, "what do you need?" or "what's up?" How negative and insensitive this sounds. It may be a sign of an unpleasant gesture. This does not motivate anyone, no matter how much you like them. Do not let it discourage you. Be courteous, sound happy, make the call short to close the conversation. End it with a warm goodbye.

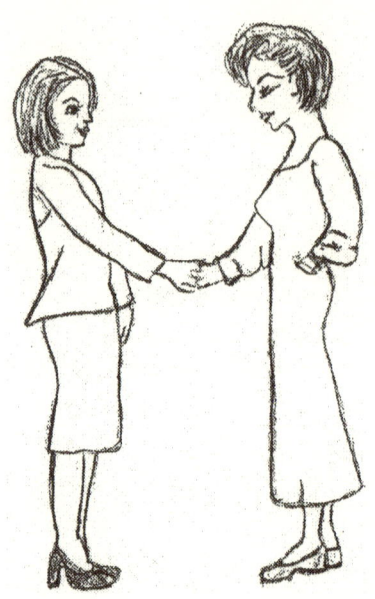

# Communication

We all learn some form of communication through our use of moral values and self-respect. Although, as we age and grow through life, we forget to practice these very special qualities, especially when we have experienced any emotional hardships.

As people get older, sometimes they become distant and unhappy, they think they know everything. My biggest reward is to possibly make a person a little kinder without trying to change anyone. Communicate verbally or with expressions. Walking with good posture projects respectful, positive body language. Take pride in all you say and do.

# TRANQUILITY

## Personal experience

I have worked all my life since the age of 16. In the various job placements I have held, I experienced and encountered unpleasant, sad, envious, and self-pity personnel. With their cold personalities, rudeness easily comes into the picture. They do not show warmth, and they hold back on caring. This could be a sign of an unpleasant upbringing, home atmosphere or personal choice. (I could be wrong). When you hold a job either at an office, hardware or department store, or any professional and employment position, your manners, or lack of them, reflect right away. Stay alert!

Many times, as children, parents or other people compare them to someone whom they hold with high regards. This hurts, that over the years this person holds unpleasant, emotional feelings and may feel frustrated. Distance can also come into the picture.

I have known beautiful women and very attractive men in my lifetime, particularly during my modeling years. The sad part is that they allow for conceit to become part of their personality and throws all that beauty and good looks out the window.

People need to show more care by being courteous, and above all, show compassion.

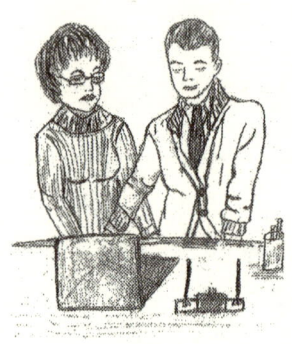

# where can I find...

## Personal skills

What kind of work skills would you like to improve? Inquire at work or at a business college for any programs or sessions to help you succeed. In case you are not into seeking a higher education, aside from a high school diploma or GED, speak with the person in charge of your department to see what you can do to better yourself in order to climb up the ladder.

How does one prepare for a position that you are highly interested in applying? Prepare yourself, by seeking information from the employees in that particular department which interests you. Check out all sources and ask the person for their job description and how it entitles them to perform other responsibilities.

Try book stores for a variety of editions on that certain subject. Make notes and affix them to your file for the vacant or upcoming position you are planning on applying. Follow your heart and trust your thinking.

# a guide

Use common sense for everyday dressing. Admiration and notice will be given to you. Love and respect yourself.

An important suggestion, when meeting people from all walks of life, give a kind and sincere greeting. Be friendly and remember your manners. Be tactful. By being tactful, is knowing what you say or do in order to have good relations with people. Let them look up to you in trust.

Be a good example in all you do!

# AFFORDABLE FASHION

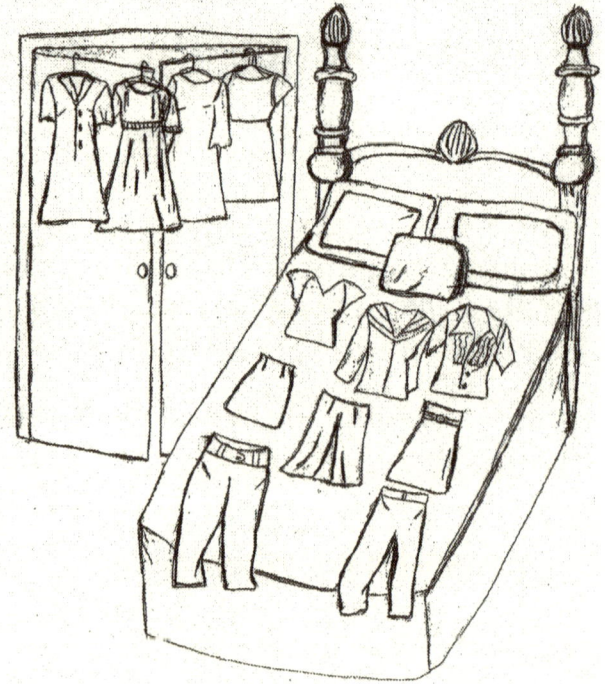

# How to dress appropriately for a job description requirement

Take your clothes from the closet and place on the bed or a clean floor, horizontal. Start with the blouses, side by side, in a row and the same with the skirts, next is the slacks. Dresses can be hung on top of a door. Take your time and combine your blouses and add to some dresses or to two (2) piece outfits. Use your imagination and picture the outfit in your mind or better yet, should you have time, put it on. Do the same with the slacks and skirts. Another suggestion is to add a larger size blouse to go over a top or dress. Do you have a variety of clothes with prints? Place them against solid pieces. Create an attractive wardrobe and trust your decision. Have fun doing this and think of the money you can save by using your common sense. Design your own style! You can look very nice with what you have on hand. Be smart and sensible, shop for basic colors. Have a pair of red flats and heels on hand for contrast with white, tan, black and navy to compliment them. Give colors spark!

Should you be more into skirts and dresses with jackets, this is great, because by removing the jacket, it will give you a different appearance for any function you may be attending. Always be ready for an unexpected event. Carry a few essentials such as face powder compact, eyeliner and lipstick. Do not forget your cologne and perfume. A fragrant lotion is always nice to wear. Whenever you shake hands with anyone, the scent will linger on their hands. A pleasant reminder of you.

Women spent a substantial amount of money on clothes, although, many women tend to have misconceptions of what colors go together, as well as, what piece to wear with each other. An outfit can look plain or maybe just hangs on a person.

Buy a fashion magazine to check out the variety of colors combined to make a striking point. Try adding jewelry, it always looks nice. Dress in mind for what the occasion calls for, be flexible and not overbearing. People will notice. Dress comfortable and decent to impress yourself and feel satisfied with your decision!

Do not lower your values or reputation.

There are a few sloppy, lazy or unmotivated people that exist and it shows how they dress. Please do not be one of them, try to help by expressing a sincere, positive comment or compliment on something that the person is wearing. For example, when the hair looks nice, tell her how it compliments her face. When she is wearing a plain dress, express how a certain color jacket would look nice. Point out an attractive face feature: smile, dimples, eyebrow, eyes. Bring to their attention a particular pair of shoes, a purse, piece of jewelry.

# DISCOVER APPRECIATION

## Job responsibility

Who is responsible for what job duties? When in a work place, everyone helps each other through team work. Do not become in the habit of thinking or saying, "This is not part of my job description". The more you learn the better the experience and perhaps even a job promotion. Keep your mind eager and anxious to learn and do. Whenever you are asked a question on a particular subject and you do not know or are not certain of an answer, let the individual know that you will inquire about it and get back to him or her. Do what you can to get any or all information. Research and play detective. Make calls, ask workers around you, and once you obtain what you need, present it and offer your assistance on anything else they may be in need of. You will portray a motivated, informative and eager to please person in the office or other surroundings.

# (brush up on your typing)

At a department store, the customer is always right, however, it may not be always true. Whatever the case may be, hear them out, express your concern with tact and patience, and reassure them that you can assist in any way possible. A content customer can make a positive comment to a manager or supervisor stating how well you assisted them. This is the best compliment anyone can receive.

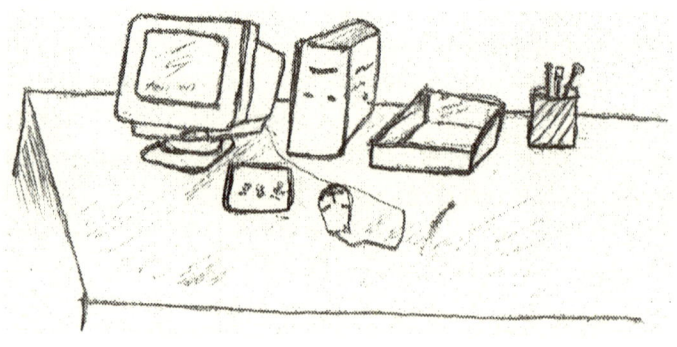

# Coordinate

## Be Organized

How you keep your desk drawer, files and office surroundings is a reflection to others of your commitment and thoroughness to a job or project. Be coordinated and jot down notes to help you remember things to do or people to assist. Be a go-getter should the need arise, and the one to keep the office, warehouse, classroom or any surrounding in a neat and organized manner. I have seen at stores, the back of computer registers full of lint, dust and papers. This says a lot of the salespeople or office workers. Since the place does not belong to them personally, why take the time and interest to dust it once in a while. Laziness can reflect a person's own negligence at their own home. This goes for both sexes. I have personally seen this at my work place and once in a while I take the initiative and clean the area.

Hiring a cleaning crew does not necessarily mean they clean well.

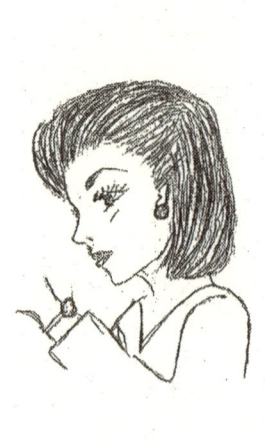

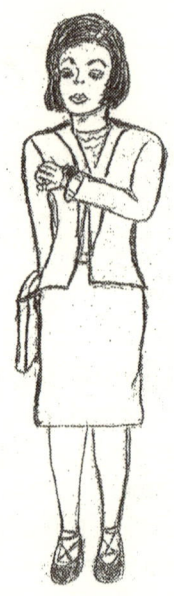

How about punctuality? What makes a person late for a commitment constantly? It can be a number of reasons or perhaps even excuses. After so many times of this irresponsible action, it becomes very frustrating and can effect any positive surrounding. Sometimes it is done intentionally to upset people. I am sure it can be embarrassing to the guilty person when someone talks to them about the situation, unless he or she is not sensitive of other people's feelings.

Take a extra step to go out of your way to please people. Do not be afraid of being taken for granted. What goes around comes around. Always smile even though the other person looks upset, it will slowly melt the frown and some how you both will feel better about the situation. Let this positive feeling radiate on your face and through your mannerism.

Love yourself and what you stand for.

# A Word
# Of Advice

# Turbulent times

I will mention rudeness again. It makes a person look ugly, even though he or she may be very attractive. This also brings a careless attitude. Fear and insecurity of expression is usually present.

(Tact is something we should all keep in mind and practice).

Many people are not fortunate to be given attention or be disciplined with care and love. It is hard for many individuals to show their feeling due to the fact that they may have been hurt, abused or neglected. It can bring out hurt in a person. Please correct it as soon as possible with dignity, courage and respect in order to continue to make good with your life. Do not be afraid to talk with the person that has caused this emotion. Also, take pride in communicating with those whom are not happy with themselves. Teach them to care. Never stop loving yourself nor feel less.

Remember, we all have our good qualities and moral values. Share your feelings of everything you know with those you love.

**PEACE OF MIND IS CLOSER THAN YOU THINK.**

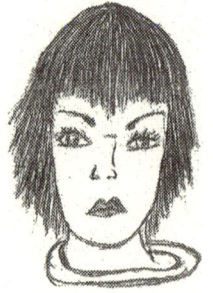

Smile and feel good within you. Your appearance will be friendly and easy going. Continue to be aware of looks, personality, character, and be responsible for your behavior with what you do and say or wherever you go.

Find happiness in your life. It is truly a wonderful feeling!

# beauty talk

## Make-up awareness

This is a wonderful subject. With so many cosmetic products on the market, it can take your breath away. I, for one, have not spent too much money on popular brand name cosmetics. Not only are they expensive, but the effect can be very similar. The ingredients also differ. Be careful with your selection. When making a decision on a particular cosmetic company, shop wisely. Be sure the company has had its products on the market for a number of years. This will ensure good quality applications. When in doubt, ask the attendant. Make it an adventure!

Eat the right foods and drink plenty of water all day long. This is one of the secrets in keeping a glowing, healthy complexion.

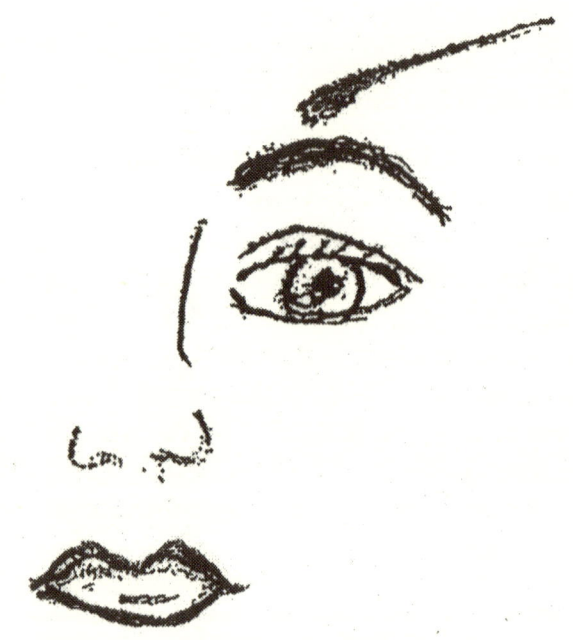

- For eyebrow: follow the natural line and fill in with soft strokes, the color as natural as your hair, when possible.

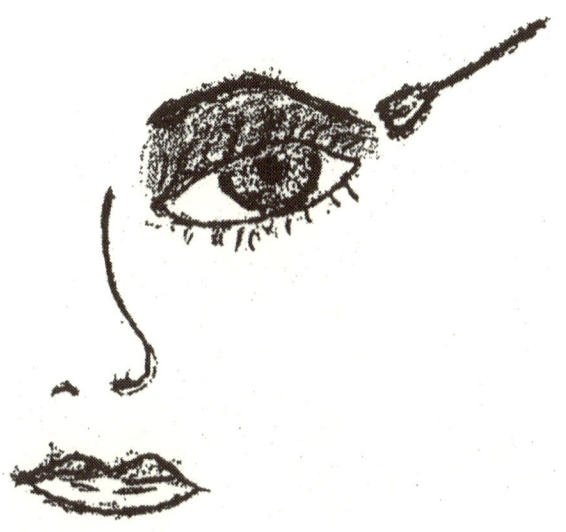

## A little hint on eye color

Before a painter can paint a new natural wood molding, he first has to prime it. This means that the first coat of paint is applied as a base or sealer followed by the actual color of paint. You can do the same. To avoid getting a crease on your eye shadow during your wearing time, gently wipe the area first with a soft cloth or tissue before the primer, which can be an off-white or natural shade of your skin color. Next, is applying your favorite eye shadow. Voila!!

P.S. I find is safer to add the eye shadow at the very beginning, before the foundation, only because some of the refine powder may accidentally fall on your face, usually the cheek bone.

You can now proceed to line the top of your eyes.

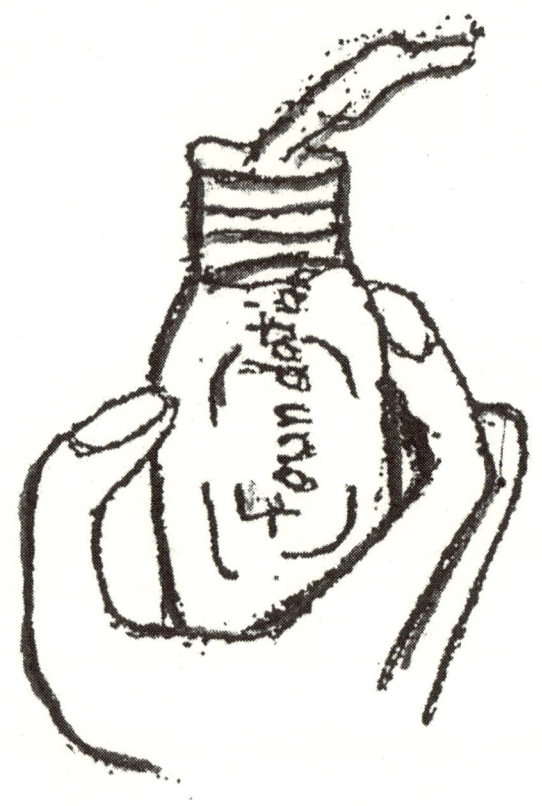

- The foundation is the liquid that is applied throughout the face for a natural tone and lightly on the neck using upward strokes.

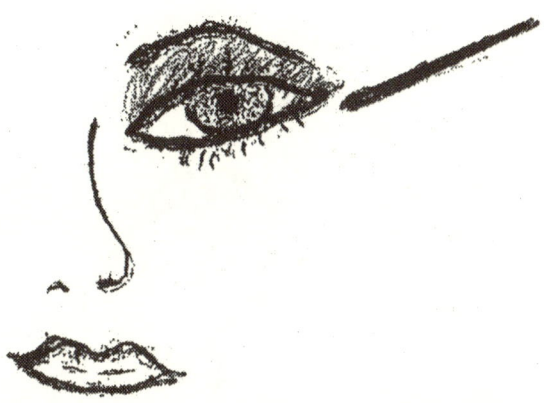

Line the bottom of your eyes after the foundation has been applied. I prefer this method. I am sure you have your own special way. Using an eyeliner is a personal preference. They come in so many colors!

The final touch is the mascara. Try to avoid using it on your lower lashes, (they do not replace themselves as quickly as your top).

This completes the eyes.

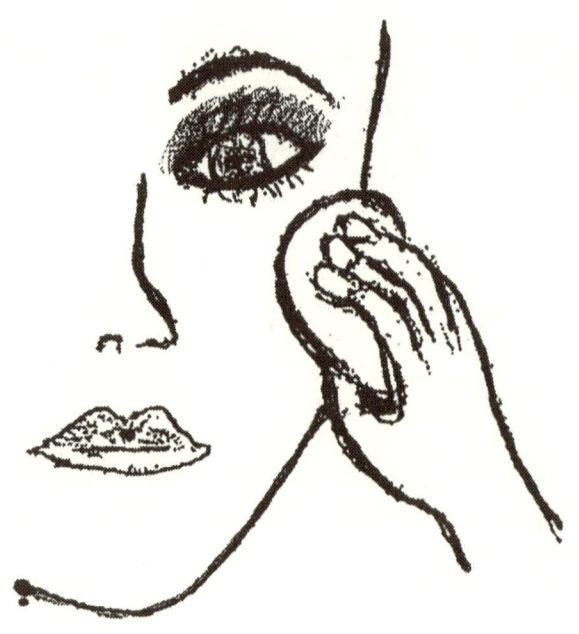

- Next is a light application of loose or compact powder to the face. A very light coat. Be sure to keep brushes and compact sponge clean at all times. You do not want to keep applying bacteria and germs to your clean face.

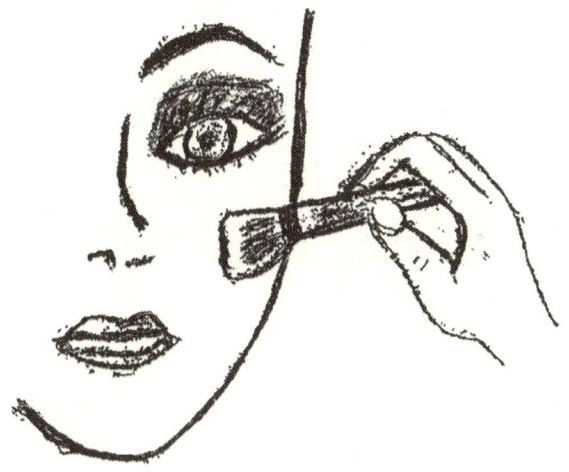

- Second to the final step for a beautiful and complete face, is the coloring or blush to the cheek bone. The shade needs to look natural. A wholesome, healthy and refreshing look.

For evening life, you may consider applying a little darker eye shadow for contrast and slightly more blush to your cheek bone. Night light has a way of deeming the face.

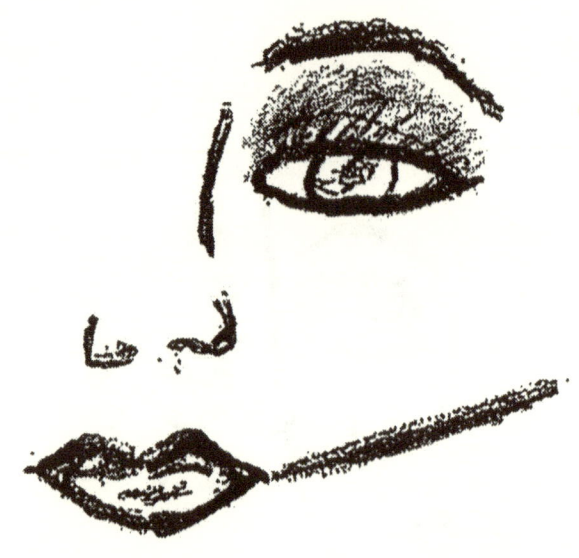

- Completion is in the lining of the lips should you decide to add it. Use a lip liner shade slightly darker than the color of your lipstick. Experiment with different colors to find your favorite one. The selection is endless.

Lipsticks vary from crèmes to shimmering shades and those that are suppose to last on longer. Choose a color that will go with your wardrobe. Should you be one to only wear neutral colors such as tan, off-white, beige, soft peach and browns, then you can stay with one color lipstick.

Wearing vibrant and vivid shades of clothing is a magical feeling for those fortunate to wear them. In this case, have a lipstick assortment.

Make your day!

I have a suggestion. It only makes sense that the makeup be removed before taking a shower or bath. Some women like baths. Are you one that enjoys showers? It is a person's preference to use cool, warm or hot water. You can lather the face with your favorite moisturing soap. When you finish rinsing yourself, be sure to splash cold water on your face, several times to close/seal the pores. (I turn the cold faucet on and only put my face into the water). This is very important for all skin types. (I do not use soap, accept for when I steam my face, once a month).

Once you dry yourself off, add your eye cream and moisturize the face.

Again, use upward strokes on your neck.

## Make up Removal

A sure way to remove your eye shadow, mascara, eyeliner, and foundation under the eyes is by using a popular brand, pure vegetable shortening. This has always worked for me. Use a soft cloth when possible and dab it off gently. Now apply the eye cream.

In case, you run out of eye makeup remover, substitute the shortening until you can replenish your own.

Use cold cream to remove the rest of your foundation, and remember, go easy on your neck. Be gentle with yourself.

# IF

A very negative word is *if.* Example: whenever you address a child to do something, a chore, for instance, a common phrase is "*if* you do not throw the trash right now, you cannot go outside, or watch TV, etc". This sounds like a threat and not very encouraging. I want to rephrase this to have a more positive approach. "I *need* you to throw the trash right now". Another example, "*when* you are finish with what you are doing, you need to throw the trash". (a child can be doing something that is important to him or her). In both instances, you will see a quick reaction from a child to this positive command. Try it!

You can also use *when* as when speaking to an adult. Example: two people are talking at some location in a building. A third person approaches them and addresses to one individual, "excuse me, *when* you finish with your conversation, I *need* to speak with you". This sounds friendly and not demanding.

Another good word is *should.* Example: this sentence is usually typed at the end of a business letter. "if you have any questions, please call me". Sounds better to read, "should you have any questions, please call me". Do you see the difference and willingness to help?

## Relaxation

People who are into aerobics, exercising, or any other form of activity, feel that this completes their overall workout. It is very important not to forget our head. What about the scalp and hair roots? There is a very simple exercise to do which benefits the head, especially the face, and helps prolong aging. Make time for yourself every day after coming home from work or school. As soon as you change out of your clothes, and into your comfortable getup, have a mat or towel handy. Spread it on the floor near a piece of furniture or the bed. Lie down and elevate your feet. No pillow! Do this for about 4 to 5 minutes. The blood will rush and circulate to your face, scalp and hair. You may feel a mild sensation and the results are fantastic. To good to be true? I dare you to try it and give it a chance. You will see results in one to two weeks. This will also relieve the pressure off your legs. While keeping your legs up, blank your mind and take a few deep breaths. You may fall asleep for a few minutes without even thinking about it. A little nap is very beneficial to all! It relaxes the body. Do your best not to frown your forehead, squint your eyes nor pout your mouth.

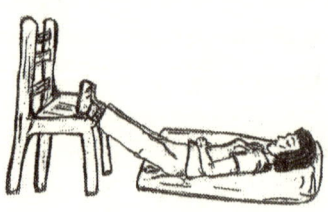

You Deserve Peace of Mind...

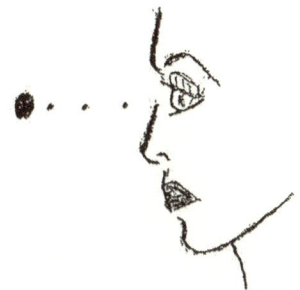

## Concentration

Exercise your eyes by focusing at a dot or any small object that may catch your attention. Relax the body and begin staring at the object. Open your eyes wide, careful not to frown your forehead. Start concentrating. Do not blink, but hold your attention as long as you possibly can at the object. Your eyes will experience a slight burning sensation. When you can no longer stand it, blink your eyes and return to your focusing. As you continue, every time you open your eyes, you will notice that for a split second, your vision will be clear. This will take about 4 to 5 times of blinking. Should you wear glasses, do it without them. This will help improve your vision. Trust me on this! Do not attempt this with contact lenses, they already have their own prescription

Hope it works for you!

## Stairs

Practice first by finding a building with stairs or perhaps be lucky to live in a two story house. No one needs to know what you are doing. After several practices and you feel comfortable about yourself, then you are ready to go out in public or social gatherings. Before you attempt to go up the stairs, wherever you may be, pause at the bottom. Place your hand on the handrail and give your first step. Keep your elbow down and close to your body with every step you take. Do not reach up by grabbing the rail to help you climb up the stairs. This makes you look tired. Keep your posture straight and knees relaxed. Continue your way to the top.

As you approach the stairs to start down, place your hand on the rail, look down with your eyes to guide you. Take your first step with your arm slightly extended and keep the elbow close by your side. This gives you a confident and graceful appearance. When descending the stairs, occasionally look down with your eyes. Keep your head up and trust yourself with each step you take. (Practice caution). Give your attention to the atmosphere at the bottom of the stairs. Do not forget to look content.

## Picking an object off the floor

As you walk and see an object or item on your path ahead of you, calculate how many steps it will take before you approach it. When you are getting close, slow your pace, and stand beside the object. Both feet are together, one foot should be slightly ahead of the other. Be sure the object is within reach. Slowly lower yourself bending the knees. The hand that is not reaching will rest on the lower thigh. The other hand will reach for the object. "Good posture is important"! Once you have the object in your hand, bring it by your side, raise yourself up slowly, using your knee muscles and keep your back straight. You can use the opposite hand that is resting on your thigh to assist in getting up. Do it easily and feel light, otherwise you may look heavy and tired. Always keep a content look on your face with whatever you do.

# F I N A L L Y...

Sometimes the good things in life really are free

I hope I have met your expectations and you feel inspired to improve yourself in one or more of the areas that were addressed. Motivation is the key to bettering yourself. Let your heart and mind work together, in order to spread everything good about yourself to the world.

I wish you happiness, joy and may all your optimum self be attained.

It's all up to you!

# Best in You!

## CLASSES

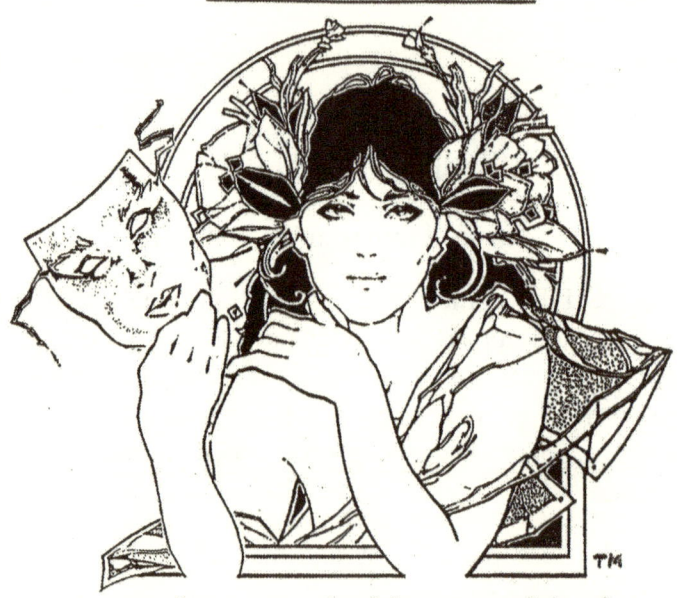

## Realize your hidden good looks

*Taught by professional model:*

## ISELA GARCIA

Isela Garcia has written, directed and produced two (2) self-improvement videos for women of all ages.

E-mail address:  iselabestinu@aol.com
Website address: http://www.best-in-u.com

P.O. Box 371701
El Paso, Texas  79937-1701
1-877/779-BEST (2378)

# God Bless America and Our Troops!!!!

# About the Author

ISELA GARCIA is a professional model and self-improvement instructor with 30 years of experience and knowledge in her field. She was the lead model for Gilbert's Women's Apparel and then studied to become an instructor at her modeling school. Over the years, she has volunteered her classes to the City of El Paso's Neighborhood Outreach Centers, Girls Detention Home and David Carrasco's Job Corps. She also judged high school beauty pageants. Her dedication to her work, with students as well as adults, has been taught with dignity, self-pride and respect.

She is the proud mother of three children, ages, 29, 31 and 33 and resides in El Paso, Texas, in the comfort of her southwestern home.